BestMedDiss

Springer awards „BestMedDiss" to the best graduate theses in medicine which have been completed at renowned universities in Germany, Austria, and Switzerland. The studies received highest marks and were recommended for publication by supervisors. They address current issues from fields of research in medicine. The series addresses practitioners as well as scientists and, in particular, offers guidance for early stage researchers.

Andreas Böhler

Collimator-Based Tracking with an Add-On Multileaf Collimator

Modification of a commercial collimator system for realtime applications

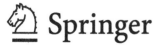 Springer

Andreas Böhler
R'n'B Medical Software Consulting GmbH
Linz, Austria

BestMedDiss
ISBN 978-3-658-10657-7   ISBN 978-3-658-10658-4 (eBook)
DOI 10.1007/978-3-658-10658-4

Library of Congress Control Number: 2015947344

Springer
© Springer Fachmedien Wiesbaden 2016

Printed on acid-free paper

Springer is a brand of Springer Fachmedien Wiesbaden
Springer Fachmedien Wiesbaden is part of Springer Science+Business Media
(www.springer.com)

Preface

The dissertation is without doubt one of the most important theses (or book!) an ongoing scientist writes throughout his career. While working on the topic is sometimes fun, sometimes frustrating and sometimes rather tedious, writing down the results is often considered boring.

It took me quite some time to push myself until I got started, but once the first few pages were there on the screen, I knew I was on the right track. A few weeks later, I had finished the first version of my thesis as a manuscript.

As usual, it took some iterations until most of the typing errors were fixed and all illustrations correctly formatted. Finally finishing my studies and being awarded the doctor's degree felt great – and I thought I was done with my dissertation.

Until almost a year later, an e-mail from my university arrived, asking if I would consent to be nominated for the Springer MedDiss 2015 programme. Of course I said "yes" without any hesitation, thinking to myself that it was an honour to be nominated, but that the chances of being actually selected for publication were not very high.

To my great delight, though, I was proven wrong, and the formatting and typesetting work started all over again – but knowing, while typing these sentences, that they would find their way into a "real" book rather soon is another good and rewarding feeling. Given the fact that a lot of dissertations end up in the university library and are never read again, this feeling is even better.

Although, at first glance, the book at hand seems rather thin, it is the result of over three years of research work. For technically-oriented work that involves a lot of software, it is sometimes hard to describe what you've done without just printing the source code.

Instead, I tried to describe on a not-too-detailed level what the main focus of the research was and how the system works in general. The first part gives an insight into the motivation of performing the work. A literature overview gives the reader the necessary knowledge of two different "worlds". On the one hand, there is the clinical background which focuses on the relevant literature. On the other hand, there is the technical background that requires a more elaborate description of the available literature and provides the reader with the necessary skills and tools to understand the concepts behind the work. The goal of the project is described briefly in chapter 3, while more attention is paid to the Materials & Methods in the following chapter. Here, the technical details of the system and the measurements performed are described. The usual section "Results" lists the insights gained and the chapters "Discussion" and "Conclusion" give a critical insight into the work.

Institution Profile

Institute for Research and Development on Advanced Radiation Technologies (radART) at the Paracelsus Medical University Salzburg

The institute was founded in 2007 (scientific head: F. Sedlmayer, administrative director: H. Deutschmann) to conduct applied research, develop technology, create methods and produce results for the advancement of treatment precision in radiotherapy. Optimized and safe healthcare solutions in the areas of medical physics, information technology, robotics, biology and radiation are being researched. Subsequently, these are implemented in patient care at the Salzburg county clinics where they are evaluated and continuously improved.

Prototypes and concepts are being developed and tested in collaboration with the medical and pharmaceutical industry. The integration of this new technology in the workflow of a clinical environment thus introduces innovations to industry and ensures that promising, new technological developments in Salzburg are widely supported by commercial partners.

The institute's priority is to be innovative in the clinical field and to ensure that prototypes, procedures and methods are developed to improve radio-therapeutic treatment of cancer patients. Thereby the Institute makes a decisive contribution to a more comprehensive use of efficient solutions in hospitals worldwide.

MedAustron

In 2012, a large-scale cooperation with the MedAustron facility was contracted, involving the development of concepts and software for the MedAustron centre built in Wiener Neustadt. MedAustron, a cancer treatment and research centre, is one of the most advanced facilities for research and ion therapy in Europe. The heart of this 200 million-euro investment, which is established and operated from the province of Lower Austria, is a particle accelerator developed in collaboration with CERN. The synchrotron (80 m ring diameter and 700 t of steel) accelerates the ions to 2/3 the speed of light and applies it precisely to the tumour.

To apply the radiation dose exactly to the tumour, a patient arrangement within millimetre precision is needed via advanced robotic patient positioning. The scientists of the radART Institute are renowned experts in this sector and provide the necessary software package to the total control of a linear accelerator in a software solution named ORA-ION. This program is derived from the institute's proprietary radiotherapy platform "open radART" (CE certified). Open radART has been developed over many years and is established in clinic mode at the University

Clinic for Radiotherapy and Radiation Oncology.

Imaging Ring

In addition, in the course of this cooperation, an innovative solution for Image guidance in photon- and ion beam therapy was designed, which is meanwhile installed at MedAustron: the so-called Imaging Ring. For construction, manufacturing and development as certified medical product, a spin-off company (Med Photon Ltd., CEO: H. Deutschmann) was founded in 2012. The unique design is based on two arms carrying X-ray source and flat panel detector mounted on a ring which is made of a highly strong aluminium-alloy. This solution, corresponding to a very light volumetric computed tomography (CT), is integrated within the patient treatment table, thus guaranteeing for utmost near-time position control prior to irradiation.

In total, the radART Institute is committed to rapid translation of scientific findings and technical developments into clinics, which is guaranteed by both: specific research focus and strong cross-linking to the Department of Radiotherapy and Radio-Oncology at the Paracelsus Medical University Clinics Salzburg.

Academic revenue is gained by publication of research results in renowned scientific journals, primarily supported by the work of students engaged within a PhD program (Dr. scient med.). The institute employs between 16 and 20 assistants and trainees, primarily IT engineers. To date, 12 doctoral theses are in preparation, another six students have already earned their doctoral degree.

Among them, Dr. Andreas Böhler's work has undoubtedly contributed to technical progress in adaptive radiotherapy, with a focus on tracking of moving targets. In a meticulous re-engineering and re-programming process, he developed a commercially available hardware device (Siemens Moduleaf), which was initially constructed for static fine conformation of field shapes only, towards a dynamic collimator, enabling real-time tracking of slowly moving tumours. Fortunately, but not surprisingly, the high quality of his dissertation was also recognized by acceptance for full-paper publication in "Physics in Medicine and Biology", one of the highest ranked scientific journals in the field.

Acknowledgements

Scientific work usually cannot be done by one person only. A number of people contributed to this, either morally, by providing valuable input or by carrying out certain tasks.

Above all, Univ.-Prof. Prim. Dr. Felix Sedlmayer provided not only valuable clinical input, but was always available for urgent questions or requests. Equally helpful by providing physical and technical input has proven Mag. Heinz Deutschmann, chief physicist, throughout the years at the institute.

Siemens OCS kindly provided background and development information about the Moduleaf system, including tools and design documents. Without their support, a re-engineering of this size wouldn't have been possible.

It is the people in the office who are responsible for a good working atmosphere. My colleagues at the radART institute provided continuous support in technical details and were always up for an interesting discussion. Furthermore, Christoph Gaisberger helped in evaluating the Gafchromic measurements while Harald Weichenberger and Markus Neuner assisted in hardware and software development work.

Last but not least I would like to thank my family. I want to especially mention my parents for offering me all the possibilities one can think of, their care and support throughout the years and their respect for all my decisions.

Thank You.

Contents

List of Figures

Abstract

Radiotherapy is one of the most important methods used for the treatment of cancer. Irradiating a moving target is also one of the most challenging tasks to accomplish in modern radiotherapy.

In this thesis, a tracking system was developed by modifying an add-on collimator, the Siemens Moduleaf, for realtime applications in radiotherapy. As the add-on collimator works almost completely autonomously of the linear accelerator (LinAc), no modifications to the latter were necessary.

The adaptations to the Moduleaf were mainly software-based. In order to reduce the complexity of the system, outdated electronic parts were replaced with newer components where practical.

Verification was performed by measuring the latency of the system as well as the impact on applied dose to a predefined target volume, moving in the leaf's travel direction.

Latency measurements in software were accomplished by comparing the target and current positions of the leaves.

For dose measurements, a Gafchromic EBT2 film was placed beneath the target 4D phantom, in between solid water plates, and moved alongside with it.

Comparing the dose distribution on the film with a moving target between "tracking disabled" towards "tracking enabled" functions resulted in penumbra widths of 23 mm to 4 mm for 0.1 Hz sinusoidal movements with an amplitude of 32 mm, respectively. The maximum speed was therefore 20 mm/s. Latency was measured to be less than 50 ms for the signal runtimes.

Based on the results, a tracking-capable add-on collimator seems to be a useful tool for reducing the margins for the treatment of small, slow-moving targets.

1. Introduction

Radiotherapy is one of the most important methods to treat cancer. Based on the tumour statistics from 2006, more than 50 % of cancer patients in the USA, Australia and the UK could benefit from the use of radiation therapy throughout their treatment (Delaney et al. 2005).

During treatments with a linear accelerator (LinAc), high energy photons are irradiated onto the human body which cause secondary electrons in human tissue. These electrons then result in DNA damage, thus destroying cells if the damage is not repaired.

In order to increase the effect on cancerous tissue, this irradiation is performed in multiple fractions, maximising the effect of different repair mechanisms in healthy tissue and tumour cells (Ahmad et al. 2012).

During external beam radiotherapy, optimal field conformation is a prerequisite for delivering curative doses to a target volume while sparing critical organs at risk (OAR).

In physical terms, this means that as much dose as possible must be applied to the tumour, but as little dose as possible has to be applied to the remaining tissue.

The introduction of MultiLeaf Collimators (MLCs) into daily routine enabled individual adaptation of treatment fields to a given shape of the target volume. Multiple, individually movable leaves shield the radiation where it is not desirable.

If the target is moving, however, organ motion may lead to a blurring of dose distributions, bearing likewise the danger of significant underdosages within the planning target volume (PTV) and overdosages in adjacent, normal tissues. The specific treatment technique is not as important as are the characteristics of the motion and the amplitude of the movement (Mzenda et al. 2010; Bortfeld, Steve B Jiang, and Rietzel 2004).

There are several strategies to apply sufficient dose to a moving target, two of them are mentioned here for comparison: The first possibility is to increase the irradiation margins, so that the tumour remains within the treatment fields throughout its entire movement (T. Inoue et al. 2013). As a consequence, however, a large amount of healthy tissue is included in the high-dose area.

Another possibility is the continuous adaptation of a treatment field to the moving target. This, however, requires the close cooperation of various subsystems, such as sensing system, control system and beam shaping tools (Geoffrey et al. 2012; Guckenberger et al. 2009; Voort van Zyp et al. 2009; Herk 2004).

As of today, only several simulations have been performed and some reference systems have been installed, investigating the use of built-in, dynamic MLCs for tracking applications. For instance, the Siemens (Siemens AG, Erlangen, Germany) 160 MLC was upgraded with tracking algorithms, using the built-in onboard kilovoltage (kV) imaging system as tracking input (Tacke et al. 2010; Krauss et al. 2012).

Another feasibility study demonstrated the use of the Varian (Varian Medical Systems, Palo Alto, USA) Millenium dynamic MLC (DMLC) in combination with an independent realtime position monitoring system for intensity modulated radiotherapy (Sawant et al. 2008; Paul J. Keall et al. 2006).

The CyberKnife system (AccuRay Inc., USA), however, is to our knowledge the only clinical implementation of a system capable of tracking moving targets (Hoogeman et al. 2009; Jereczek-Fossa et al. 2013).

In this thesis, a system using an add-on MLC to dynamically adapt the shape of the beam to changed conditions is presented. This device works almost completely autonomously, without interfering with the LinAc, which, therefore, does not need to be modified.

2. Literature Overview

2.1. Introduction

As already explained in chapter 1, optimal field conformation throughout the entire radiotherapeutic treatment is of utmost importance. In the case of a moving target organ, special care has to be taken.

The first section therefore deals with the clinical literature and tries to give an insight into the motivation of developing the system.

Besides the clinical motivation of optimal patient treatment, there are also technical aspects to consider. Developing realtime control systems and being able to control a great number of independently moving leaves is not only a challenging, but also a very interesting and demanding task. Thus, the second part of the literature overview deals with the technical details of this work.

2.2. Clinical Literature

Current radiation therapy treatment techniques focus on accurate and fast dose delivery. For instance, image guided radiotherapy (IGRT) maximises treatment accuracy by acquiring images of the treatment area right before the actual irradiation is performed. Onboard kV imaging systems can be used to accomplish this task. Intensity modulated radiotherapy (IMRT) uses a great amount of very small, irregularily shaped fields (in the case of step-and-shoot IMRT) to achieve very steep gradients and non-uniform dose distributions within a single field.

Modern IMRT treatments are not made up of a limited number of small fields, but of continuously adapted fields using a dynamic MLC (DMLC) (McMahon, Papiez, and Rangaraj 2007; Poulsen, Cho, Sawant, and Paul J Keall 2010; Falk et al. 2010).

Stereotactic radiotherapy is used where accuracy matters most: For the treatment of brain tumours, for example, additional steps like fixating the patient's head are performed (Ahmad et al. 2012; Ikushima 2010).

Due to physiological factors, such as respiration or organ motion, some tumours attached to or in proximity of the respective organ can be in continuous or partial movement throughout the irradiation. This motion may result in a blurring of the dose distribution and can cause interplay effects in the case of IMRT treatments (Bortfeld, Steve B Jiang, and Rietzel 2004).

Usually, the movement of a tumour is not only in the horizontal plane, but also in other dimensions. Recently, some efforts have been put in developing tracking algorithms for calculating the optimal leave positions for tumours moving in 3D space. These algorithms require a DMLC, which then executes the calculated movements (Sawant et al. 2008; Trofimov et al. 2008).

Such dynamic MLCs have been integrated into, e.g., the Siemens 160-MLC, which was equipped with a modified control system and image-based tracking input. Due to the latency of >400 ms, dosimetric accuracy was limited (Tacke et al. 2010; Krauss et al. 2012).

For a DMLC, a few parameters are important that characterise and influence the system's ability to follow (track) a moving target: accuracy and system latency.

Accuracy is defined as the overall difference between target position and current position i.e. the geometrical error. System latency, on the other hand, is defined as the time lag the tracking control system introduces.

For current DMLC implementations, tracking accuracy and system latency vary widely: From 160 ms to over 400 ms for the latency and from 0.6 mm to 1.1 mm for the geometrical accuracy (Tacke et al. 2010; Paul J. Keall et al. 2006).

But as important the characteristics of the DMLC are concerning tracking performance, equally important is the influence of tracking inputs. Currently, several different systems are available making use of either image based systems using the onboard kV system or mechanical systems like respiratory belts. Other systems include surface scanning techniques using devices such as video projectors or cameras to detect the movement. While image-based systems, limited by the speed of the X-Ray system, introduce a relatively high latency of >400 ms, respiratory tumour tracking systems, for example, reduce the latency to <200 ms (Tacke et al. 2010; Hoogeman et al. 2009; Gaisberger et al. 2013).

Another method to cope with moving targets is the use of gating systems. In this approach, the motion tracking system decides whether the tumour is currently within the treatment field and instructs the LinAc to release the beam. As soon as the tumour moves out of the treatment field, the irradiation is suppressed (Steve B. Jiang 2006; Vedam et al. 2001; Kubo and Hill 1996).

The patient can also be instructed to hold his breath, thus reducing motion due to respiration. This is called Deep Inspiration Breath Hold (DIBH) technique (Mageras and Yorke 2004).

2.3. Technical Literature

Measuring 6 MV photon beams, for instance for quality control or routine checks, can be performed using several strategies, involving the use of either ionisation chambers, diodes or radiochromic films (Knoll 2010).

All measurement techniques differ in the way they are performed and their practical use. Ionisation chambers deliver very good energy responses, but accumulate dose over a larger area and can thus not reflect steep gradients (penumbras), used for example in IMRT treatments. Diodes and diode arrays, on the other hand, feature a smaller active detector area and smaller volume and are therefore better suited for steep gradients. Radiochromic films, such as the Gafchromic EBT2 film can be used on a wide range of energies for use in radiotherapy. The advantage of this type of film is its self developing nature. This means that the irradiated areas are visible with bare eyes. On the downside, it requires calibration for every batch as well as a calibrated scanner and lookup tables for absolute dosimetry (Laub and Wong 2003; Paliwal and Tewatia 2009; Butson et al. 2010; Cheung, Butson, and Yu 2006; García-Garduño et al. 2008; Arjomandy et al. 2012).

For the creation of these lookup tables, until recently only the red channel was chosen, as it provides good linearity over a wide dose range. Newer methods suggest the use of triple channel calibration to increase accuracy of the radiochromic film even further (Hayashi et al. 2012).

Apart from the measurement of dose and dose distributions, DMLC systems, consisting of up to 160 independently moving leaves, require control systems being able to keep all leaves in coordinated movement. There are several factors that influence the performance of such a system, for instance the design of the individual leaves and the mechanical drive system. Of equal importance are the leaf position detection, the transmission of positional information and the control loops themselves (Boyer et al. n.d.).

2.3.1. Multileaf Collimator

The MLC consists of a number of leaves, made of beam shielding material such as tungsten, that can be moved independently in order to adapt the shape of the treatment field to the actual tumour volume.

Figure 2.1 graphically illustrates the principle of a multileaf collimator with 18 leaves shown.

2.3.2. Design of Individual Leaves

The individual leaf may be designed in a way that it can travel to a certain degree beyond the centre line of the MLC (overtravel; in figure 2.1, leaves 101, 102, 108 and 109 are in an overtravel position). The amount of overtravel depends on the actual MLC manufacturer: the Elekta MLC leaves can overtravel up to 10 cm for the pre-Agility MLC (MLCi), while the Moduleaf miniMLC leaves are capable of

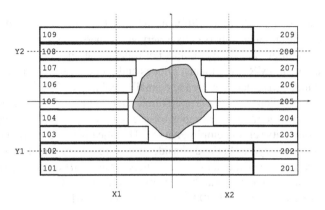

Figure 2.1: Graphical illustration of a multileaf collimator; only 9 leaf pairs are shown; Image by ZEEs under GFDL.

nearly full overtravel (55 mm overtravel compared to a total field length of 120 mm) (Boyer et al. n.d.; Crop et al. 2007).

Several leaves together may then be fixed on a moving block, so that the complete leaf bank can be moved as well, thus increasing the length of overtravel. This design is used in the Varian MLCs and the newer Elekta Agility MLCs (Boyer et al. n.d.; Bedford, Thomas, and Smyth 2013).

Usually, one DC motor per leaf is used to drive it to the desired position. The type of motor and its characteristics are responsible for the speed of the leaf. Typical speeds range from 0.2 mm/s to 50 mm/s (Boyer et al. n.d.).

2.3.3. Leaf Position Detection and Data Transfer

Another characteristic of an MLC is the way the actual position of a leaf is determined. This detection is necessary for the control loops to drive a leaf to its desired position. For safety purposes, more than one way of determining the position may be used.

Video-optical systems, such as those in use by Elekta, require a light source, reflective material at each leaf end and a camera to detect the reflections. The advantages of this system are little space and wiring requirements inside the collimator head. On the other hand, frequent camera replacement is required, as the camera is sensitive to radiation damages (Boyer et al. n.d.).

Another possibility to read the positional information are high-precision linear potentiometer systems, as used by, e.g., the Siemens Moduleaf. Potentiometers are technically easy to read, but accuracy and linear range are often in conflict. Thus, two potentiometers can be combined to gain the advantages of both potentiometers or for verification purposes (one potentiometer verifies the position of the other). A disadvantage are the space and wiring requirements inside the head, as each potentiometer requires separate wiring (Boyer et al. n.d.; Crop et al. 2007).

For special, binary MLCs, e.g. the Tomotherapy system, simple limit switches can give feedback on the binary position of the leaf (Boyer et al. n.d.; Mackie et al. 1999).

After having measured the positions of the leaves, these values need to be transferred to the control system. For camera-based systems, this could be achieved in analogue form by using a coaxical cable. For digital systems, such as the Moduleaf, it is common to use bus-based systems in conjunction with controllers near the motor, to reduce the number of required cables.

The Controller Area Network (CAN) bus, although having been developed in the 1980's by Bosch (Robert Bosch GmbH, Gerlingen-Schillerhöhe, Germany), is still widely used in automation tasks and cars. Thanks to its design, it can be used for realtime applications in various scenarios and is common in medical applications (Tindell, Hansson, and Wellings 1994; Farsi and Ratcliff 1997; Farsi, Ratcliff, and Barbosa 1999a; Pinho and Vasques 2003; Farsi, Ratcliff, and Barbosa 1999b; Yime 2008).

Based on twisted-pair cables, the bus can be up to 100 m long, with the maximum baud rate of 1 Mbit/s up to 40 m are possible. On top of the Data Link Layer, which uses a CSMA/CA algorithm, a number of high level protocols can be implemented.

CSMA/CA is the abbreviation for Carrier Sense Multiple Access with Collision Avoidance and describes the possibility of several nodes (Multiple Access) to "listen" for activity on the bus (Carrier Sense) and to avoid frame collision (Collision Avoidance) by only transmitting data when no other node is currently transferring. If a collision occurs, the higher priority node transmits first (Ziouva and Antonakopoulos 2002; Pfeiffer, Ayre, and Keydel 2008).

CANopen is one example of such a high level protocol, featuring not only profiles for various types of CAN nodes, but also providing capabilities for monitoring nodes and implementing state machines. Different message types with different functionalities are defined: service data objects (SDO) and process data objects (PDO).

A drawback of CANopen is the relatively high protocol overhead for SDO messages (4 bytes), compared to the small data payload of only 8 bytes per CAN message frame. As a result, PDO messages can be used to stream data more efficiently (all 8 data bytes available), but require a preceeding SDO message for

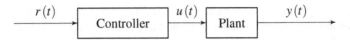

Figure 2.2: Open Loop control system. The input r is used by the Controller to control the plant, but without providing feedback.

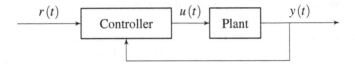

Figure 2.3: Closed Loop control system. The input r is used by the Controller to control the plant, including feedback.

the initiation of the transfer (Pfeiffer, Ayre, and Keydel 2008; Cena and Valenzano 2003).

2.3.4. Control System and Control Loops

A microprocessor system, be it a microcontroller platform or an industrial computer or a workstation, has to "digest" all given inputs and has to decide how fast and how far to drive the leaf so that it reaches its target position.

For this purpose, Control Loops are used which permanently compare target and current positions, incorporate a feedback loop (for closed loop systems) and decide on the output. In figure 2.2 an open loop, in figure 2.3 a closed loop are shown for comparison. While the open loop does not provide any feedback, the closed loop takes the actual position into consideration.

Several standard-based control loops exist, which can also be combined. The literature distinguishes between various standard elements, such as the proportional, the integral and the derivative controller. For the following sections, the symbol $y(t)$ is used to describe the controller's output, $u(t)$ describes the actuator signal, $r(t)$ the reference input and K_P, K_I and K_D are the respective weighing factors.

The proportional element, abbreviated as "P", is only a gain onto the input signal. Its step response is thus the original signal multiplied by the gain, K_P.

$$y(t) = K_P u(t) \tag{2.1}$$

The integral element, abbreviated as "I", is basically an integrator, which

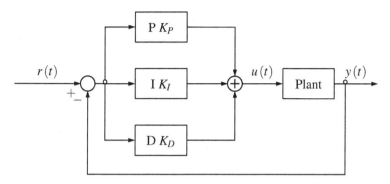

Figure 2.4: Overview of a PID controller

integrates the input signal over time. Its weighing factor is given by K_I.

$$y(t) = K_I \int u(t)\, dt \qquad (2.2)$$

The derivative element, abbreviated as "D", derivates the input signal. Its weighing factor is given by K_D.

$$y(t) = K_D \frac{du(t)}{dt} \qquad (2.3)$$

These three basic elements can be combined differently, so that PI, PD or PID controllers are possible. The respective factor determines the weight of each element and has significant influence on the outcome. The complete equation for a PID controller in time domain is

$$y(t) = K_P u(t) + K_I \int u(t)\, dt + K_D \frac{du(t)}{dt} \qquad (2.4)$$

while the block diagram of a PID controller is shown in figure 2.4 (Åström and Hägglund 2001). PID controllers are very robust and can be used for a variety of applications, but are not the ideal choice for unstable, resonant or integrating processes (Atherton and Majhi 1999).

If every element of the control system is known in detail, including models of the motor and the mechanical construction, the optimum values for the control loop can be calculated. By the term "optimum" a combination of parameters is described that fulfils certain criteria like overshoot, stability, etc. (Liu and Daley 2001).

If not every value is known, however, empirical methods, such as the Ziegler-Nichols method, can be used to find the optimal parameters. This method involves the individual adjustment of each parameter online until the system begins to oscillate. Then, the value being adjusted is decreased to find a stable state again (Åström and Hägglund 1995; Åström and Hägglund 2004).

Usually, the Ziegler-Nichols method gives a steep response with some overshoot involved, resulting from aggressive values for the gain (the "P" controller) and only small values for the "I" and "D" parts in order to minimise the effects of gain and overshoot (Åström and Hägglund 1995).

3. Hypothesis & Goals

The university clinic for radiotherapy and radio-oncology in Salzburg/Austria has been using a Moduleaf miniMLC for several years for clinical applications. The department is equipped with Elekta linear accelerators, to which the miniMLC is nearly fully compatible. During routine treatments, usually stereotactic irradiations on small tumours are performed. Due to the design and age of the Moduleaf miniMLC, its use is restricted to these radiosurgical applications, but current treatment techniques such as dynamic IMRT treatments or tracking applications are not possible.

In the course of this work a control system shall be implemented for the Moduleaf miniMLC that features tight integration into the open source Record and Verify system open radART (medPhoton GmbH, Salzburg, Austria). The primary goal of this control system are tracking applications, but the system's input shall be generic enough for, e.g., dynamic IMRT treatments.

Further, the dosimetric impact of the system has to be evaluated as well as if and to what degree the newly developed system can be clinically used. For this purpose, a test setup using a 4D phantom has to be designed. A corresponding evaluation system has to be set up and worked on as well.

Gaining knowledge about the current tumour position, the tracking input signal, is not part of this work. Several other systems can be used for this task, an overview is given in section 2.2.

4. Materials & Methods

The university clinic's second Moduleaf miniMLC unit, currently not in clinical use, was taken as a development platform. Together with some spare parts and electronics obtained with the help of Siemens, a complete development environment was set up.

This chapter is split into several sections, which give an overview on how the development process was implemented and what tools are required. Furthermore, the test setup and data analysis tools are explained in detail.

4.1. Hardware

The Moduleaf, originally developed by MRC Systems GmbH/Germany consists of 80 leaves with a leaf width of 2.5 mm in the isocentre. It therefore matches conformation needs also for the majority of brain stereotactic treatments (Wu et al. 2009). When mounted on an Elekta (Elekta AB, Stockholm, Sweden) LinAc, it is rotated by 90° with regard to the integrated MLC. The maximum leaf travel speed is 30 mm/s in the isocentre (Schlegel et al. 2006).

By original design, only step and shoot IMRT treatments are possible. The collimator control system simply cuts power to the motors once a given position has been reached. Rotational treatments, VMAT/RapidArc or tracking are therefore impossible in the original implementation. Being a clear limitation, efforts were taken to re-engineer parts of the commercial system.

In its original configuration, the Moduleaf consists of a number of hardware parts that communicate with each other. This communication is outlined in figure 4.1.

The control computer is a Pentium III class standard desktop PC in a custom housing, equipped with 128 MB of random access memory (RAM). One of the ISA slots, however, is equipped with a SORCUS (SORCUS Computer GmbH, Heidelberg, Germany) ML-4 single board computer (SBC), including modules for the Controller Area Network (CAN) bus and digital input/output (DIO).

The CAN-bus is then connected via a multi-core cable, where also power and interlock signals are transmitted, to the collimator itself. Inside the carbonium casing, 6 C167CR (Infineon Technologies AG, Munich, Germany) microcontrollers are attached to the CAN bus. Each of them controls up to 16 leaves and has several interlock lines connected to the control system as well.

Given the age of the system, several components such as ISA bus single board computers are not produced anymore and do not provide the necessary data through-

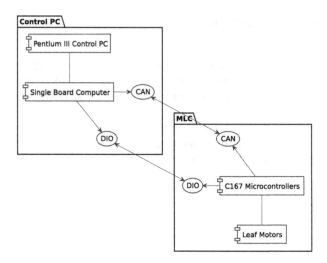

Figure 4.1: Original implementation; the Single Board Computer is connected to the microcontroller system and responsible for safety monitoring

put for realtime applications. Thus, those components were either removed or replaced by newer systems.

Figure 4.2 (Böhler et al. 2015) visualises the interplay of the updated components. The C167CR microcontrollers were left in place, but communicate directly via CAN with the control computer. The intermediate single board computer is completely removed and its functionality is now incorporated into other subsystems.

SORCUS's real-time operating system on the ML-4 acted for one part as a bridge between the control computer and the CAN bus. Being an intelligent component, it also supervised the information flow on the CAN message level, but also on the Interlock line level. Thus, only if all microcontrollers reported a healthy state, the LinAc's interlock was released. The last functionality of this SBC is therefore the communication with the LinAc, depending on the configuration using only Interlock lines or more advanced systems like the CAN bus for tighter integration.

The supervision of the CAN message flow is now incorporated into the control application on the control computer itself, while the interlock supervision requires an external system. This additional safety controller, which also communicates with the LinAc, is explained in more detail in section 4.1.2.

Some of the important components along with their characteristics are presented

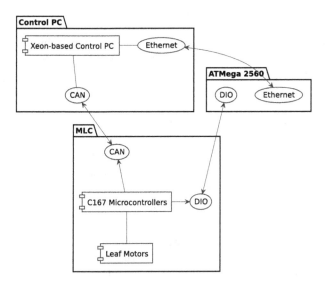

Figure 4.2: New implementation; the control computer is directly attached to the microcontroller system and an additional microcontroller is responsible for safety monitoring in the following subsections.

4.1.1. C167CR microcontroller

The Infineon C167CR microcontroller units (MCUs), already present in the commercial design, were not modified in terms of hardware components. However, they play a key role in both old and new software designs as they directly control the movement of the leaves. The C167 family is binary-compatible to the older C166 MCU. This particular variant, the C167CR-LM 16-bit MCU, is clocked at 20 MHz, features 2 kB internal RAM for variables, register banks, system stack and code as well as another 2 kB of XRAM, which can be used for variables, user stack and code, too. A key feature of this microcontroller is the interrupt system that provides 56 interrupt nodes which can be configured in 16 different priority levels. Directly on the chip are two 16-channel capture/compare units, four 16-bit timers/counters and a 4-channel pulse width modulation (PWM) unit. Furthermore, there are five additional general-purpose timers/counters, an asynchronous/synchronous serial channel unit (USART), a 10-bit 16-channel analogue/digital (AD) converter and a CAN bus module. 111 input/output (IO) lines with individual bit addressability are available for additional input and output tasks.

An external CAN transceiver is connected to the CAN bus controller that provides access to the physical layer of the CAN bus. This device is configured so that it receives only messages that match the microcontroller's CAN ID (message mask). It raises an interrupt whenever a message is ready for retrieval, eliminating the need to constantly poll for new messages.

To control the motors, up to 16 motor drivers are connected to the IO lines of the microcontrollers. The drivers require a pulse width modulated (PWM) signal that directly corresponds to the speed of the motor. The PWM signal is not generated by the on-board PWM units, but rather by using the interrupt subsystem for practical reasons.

Since each leaf has two high-precision potentiometers attached that can be used to read the current position, AD converters are necessary. Because of the high precision requirements, the onboard AD converter is unused. Instead, an external 16-bit AD converter is connected to the IO lines. As there are up to 16 leaves, two 16-channel multiplexers and one two-channel multiplexer are attached as well. This way, up to 32 potentiometers can be read one after the other with a single AD converter.

A number of light emitting diodes (LEDs) that report system states and two interlock lines are attached to the digital IOs as well.

4.1.2. Safety microcontroller

As mentioned before, another way of supervising the interlock lines and communicating with the LinAc had to be found after the removal of the SBC. Being aware of rapid prototyping platforms, the Arduino open source platform was chosen for this purpose. On the selected model, the Arduino Mega2560, an Atmel (Atmel Corporation, San Jose, USA) ATMega2560 8-bit microcontroller is present. In this case, the MCU operates at 16 MHz, provides 54 IO lines, 8 kB of RAM and 256 kB of Flash ROM for storing user code. A 10-bit AD converter is provided, which is multiplexed on 16 channels. Four hardware USART units can be used for input and output, as well as the serial peripheral interface (SPI) bus for communication with external peripherals.

For communication with the control computer, the Arduino Ethernet Shield was put in place. It uses a WIZnet (WIZNET, Hwangsaeul-ro, Bundang-gu, Seongnam-si, Gyeonggi-do, South Korea) W5100 ethernet controller, connected by SPI to the ATMega MCU. The WIZnet ethernet interface is a 100 Mbit ethernet controller that incorporates the TCP/IP stack on-chip, offloading the TCP/IP protocol handling from the MCU to this dedicated chip. Up to four simultaneous socket connections are supported, an interrupt signals the ATMega the arrival of new data.

The Arduino's IO lines were connected to the MLC hardware and the LinAc, respectively. It is in charge of resetting the MLC MCUs, supervising the interlock lines, controlling power to the DC motors and signalling the LinAc when to release and when to inhibit the beam.

4.1.3. Control Computer

The new design relocates a lot of the processing power required to control the movements of the DC motors to the control application. Furthermore, adaptations to the treatment field are done on-line, while the beam is on. Therefore, a powerful machine is necessary that can handle these tasks without being at its limit. A current Intel Quad-Core Xeon machine equipped with 4 GB of RAM and two Gigabit ethernet cards was installed instead of the old control machine.

Using the first ethernet interface, communication with the safety MCU is performed, while the second ethernet interface provides an uplink to the hospital network.

Communication with the MLC MCU subsystem is realised via a Peripheral Component Interconnect (PCI) CAN controller, as explained in the following section 4.1.4.

4.1.4. Softing PCI-CAN interface

In order to give the control computer access to and direct control over the CAN
bus, a dedicated PCI CAN controller was installed. This Softing (Softing AG, Haar,
Germany) CAN-AC2 controller features two CAN channels and is fully compliant
with the CAN bus specification. Drivers are provided for a wide range of Windows
operating systems, as well as for Linux.

4.2. Software

All these new hardware and electronical components cannot operate without software. The main development work was put into the software part, as a lot of
hardware components were readily available and seemed to be sufficient to reach
the goal. This section therefore details the development environment, MCU software, control software and control loops.

4.2.1. Development Environment

The Moduleaf's original software was implemented using a number of different
tools. The C167 MCU firmware was written using the Keil (Keil, Munich, Germany)
development tools for C166. In order to programme the SBC, Borland (Borland
Software Corporation, Austin, USA) C Compiler 3.1 for DOS was used. The
control computer's software is implemented using an ActiveX component in C++
as well as a graphical user interface (GUI) written in VisualBasic. Several external
libraries are necessary to provide treatment plan import/export capabilites and
communication interfaces to the LinAc.

The changed hardware requires a different software environment and was
updated to current technologies. Therefore, the C167 MCU firmware was reim-
plemented using the Altium Tasking VX-toolset (Altium, Belrose, Australia) for
C166 [1], after initial trials with the free and now defunct HighTec GNU compiler
toolchain did not succeed.

Development for the Arduino platform, despite the availability of the Arduino
integrated development environment (IDE), was done using the Qt Creator IDE [2]
and the avr-gcc[3] toolchain.

Qt Creator was also used for the development of the control computer's software,

---

[1]http://www.tasking.com/products/c166/, accessed Jan 2014

[2]http://qt-project.org, accessed Jan 2014

[3]http://gcc.gnu.org/wiki/avr-gcc, accessed Jan 2014

with the GCC toolchain[4] under the hood.

The primary develoment platform was based on Ubuntu[5]/GNU Linux 10.04 and 12.04, respectively. The Tasking toolchain requires Microsoft Windows, a dedicated virtual Windows XP environment was used for this purpose.

The development environment is built on free software wherever possible. Unfortunately, there is no free (free as in "free speech", not free as in "free beer") toolchain for the C167 family of microcontrollers available. Thus, the next best alternative was the use of HighTec's C166 compiler, which is at least freely available upon request from the developer (free as in "free beer"). As this compiler led to random crashes of the MCU, the same code was recompiled using Altium's Tasking compiler and now works reliably.

4.2.2. Microcontroller Firmware

The re-engineering of the MLC MCU firmware was one of the main development tasks in order to reach the goal of a tracking capable control system. Initially, it was investigated to what extent the commercial firmware could be used and if a rewrite was necessary. The first idea was thus to use the existing commandset for the SBC to MLC MCU communication and implement a pseudo-tracking system. For this purpose, up to 100 treatment fields were pre-calculated on the control computer an then transferred to the MCU system. Using a Python evaluation software, it was found that the latency of >300 ms led to uncertainties in the current positions. Furthermore, the leaves were not speed controlled, thus differences of up to 10 mm were found for a travel range of 100 mm (all values in the isocentre). The transfer of a single field to the MLC MCU system took 1.1 s, for 100 fields this is more than 1 min. The way positional information is transferred and the requirement for polling the MCU system for information were identified as limiting factors.

Based on these initial trials, it was decided to re-engineer the complete firmware and the way positional information is transferred. After initialising the system, consisting of the MCU system initialisation and the configuration via the CAN bus, the MCU system uses a hardware timer (Timer 3) unit to read the values from the potentiometers. Every 20 ms, this timer fires and the following sequence is run:

1. Set variable axis number to 1 and start a loop from axis 1 to axis 16

2. Set the first mulitplexer to the given axis

---

[4]http://gcc.gnu.org, accessed Jan 2014
[5]http://www.ubuntu.com, accessed Jan 2014

3. Read from the external ADC and store it as Potentiometer 1 value for the given axis

4. Set the second multiplexer to the second potentiometer system

5. Read from the external ADC and store it as Potentiometer 2 value for the given axis

6. Run one iteration of the Control Loop for the given axis

7. Set the second multiplexer to the first potentiometer system

8. Increase the axis number by one and start over

In order to be compatible with the original control software, the configuration can be changed, so that the MCU system must be polled for positional information. The control loop that is run in step 6 differentiates between the available modes. In Host Loop Mode, the newly developed operating mode, no actual control loop is run on the MLC MCU system. Rather, every 4 axes one CAN message is sent to the control computer containing the raw position values from the ADC system. Contrary to the commercial implementation, no conversion of ADC units of any kind is performed on the MCU level. This work is offloaded to the control application. Also, no filtering, smoothing or other data processing is performed on the MCU in this mode.

Upon arrival of a new target position via the CAN bus, an interrupt one level lower than the interrupt used for AD conversion is raised. This interrupt causes the CAN message handler to set a new PWM output value to the PWM generation system.

The PWM generation system itself does not use the hardware PWM units, but a software implementation for practical reasons. The C167CR features special capture/compare (CAPCOM) units, that can toggle an output when the CAPCOM unit overflows. Therefore, only the correct CAPCOM value for overflow has to be written to a register, the remaining output toggling is handled by the C167 hardware system. This makes software-based PWM generation very efficient.

When the MCU is idle, verification and plausibility checks are performed. For this purpose, the values of the two potentiometer systems are compared. If they are not within a certain, configurable range, the MCU's interlock is raised, causing a reaction by the safety controller.

In standard PID loop mode, when the commercial control software is used, the workflow differs. In this case, there is an actual PID control loop run on the MLC MCU system. Raw ADC values are also smoothed using a simple finite impulse response (FIR) filter, averaging the last three values. This implementation ensures that the control loop is run at fixed intervals, with a period length of 20 ms.

4.2.3. Control Software

The control software on the control computer has several functionalities and is thus split into libraries, threads and logical blocks.

If the signal flow from the MCU unit is followed, new positional information arrives via the CAN bus on the PCI CAN interface. There is an open source interface driver provided by Softing, which gives the programmer access to the CAN bus. Using this API, a software library, libCOSMICrtcan, was written that provides a hardware abstraction layer (HAL) for the higher level control system.

4.2.3.1. libCOSMICrtcan

This HAL is based on the API provided by Softing and the Boost [6] C++ library. The latter is used to ease thread programming and cross-thread communication using Mutexes and Queues. Being a HAL, the library can be forced into simulation mode or, if no actual CAN controller is found, turns on simulation mode automatically. In simulation mode, the MLC MCU system can be talked to as usual, but the communication is simulated at the library level. Every CAN message sent to the MLC MCU system in this mode is reacted upon by the library. This method provides easy debugging and testing scenarios without the need to access the MLC hardware. However, no physical simulation is performed. This means that the positional feedback is based on timers only and no characteristics such as acceleration/deceleration effects, drive systems or signal runtimes are taken into account.

The use of this library is also important for portability reasons. In order to run the control system under Microsoft Windows, mainly this library needs to be adapted to the Windows driver provided by Softing. The reamining parts of the control application only use cross-platform toolkits and thus should be already compatible with Windows, too.

4.2.3.2. COSMICrt

Being the main control application, COSMICrt has great responsibility and a number of parallel tasks to accomplish. Its name, however, is based on the commercial application's name, COSMIC, which is an acronym for "Control System for Multileaf Collimators". The added suffix "rt" signals its realtime capabilities.

To better understand and explain the information flow within the application,

---

[6]http://www.boost.org, accessed Jan 2014

a flowchart is shown in figure 4.3. Upon startup of the application, the software itself is initialised and the configuration database is parsed. This SQLite[7] database contains information about the various tracking features, calibration data for the leaves and for the 4D phantom, etc.

Initially, this configuration can be imported from the commercial implementation's calibration file, mlc70.ini. As calibrating the system involves manual measurements using a slide gauge, it is a very tedious task that can be shared with the clinical application very easily.

Afterwards, 5 threads are initialised, each having a very specific duty.

Safety Thread It is responsible for communicating with the safety MCU. If all leaf positions are within tolerance, the LinAc is released.

Phantom Thread Its duty is the reading of the current 4D phantom positions and the calculation of the new target positions.

CAN Thread This is the most important thread as it communicates with the MLC MCUs, reads the current positions, runs the control loops and sets new PWM output values to the MLC hardware.

Governor Thread Also in communication with the safety thread, the Governor Thread constantly checks the current and target position deviation and signals the safety thread when and if the system is in or out of tolerance.

GUI Thread It is responsible for visualising the state of the software and for accepting user input.

When an irradiation is to be performed, the workflow is as follows: The record & verify system (PRVS), for instance open radART (medPhoton GmbH, Salzburg, Austria), sends a request including the field definition to the COSMICrt software. The treatment field is loaded, visualised and the leaves are brought into the initial position. When performing a tracked treatment, the tracking system must be initialised and COSMICrt told where to receive the inputs from. From now on, the treatment field is constantly adapted to the new positions of the tumour as reported by the external system.

The main interface of COSMICrt also displays a realtime graph showing the tracking target positional variations over time. The radiotherapist can use this display to verify the movements of the tumour.

---

[7]SQLite is a software library that implements a self-contained, serverless, zero-configuration, transactional SQL database engine; http://www.sqlite.org, accessed Jan 2014

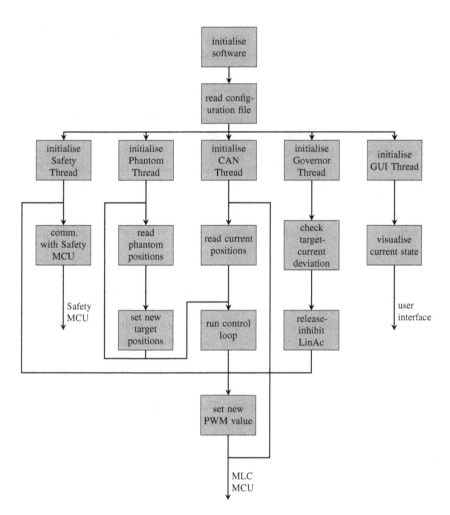

Figure 4.3: Overview of software information flow

A screenshot of the control interface is shown in figure 4.4 (Böhler et al. 2015). Here, the MLC target positions are visualised in grey while the current MLC positions are shown in blue. This screenshot was taken during positioning, some leaves have already reached their target positions while others are still moving.

If no connection to an external PRVS is available, field shapes can also be imported from local files. The format of COSMICrt fields is based on the extensible markup language (XML) and contains descriptions of the various leaf settings. In order to import plan files from open radART, a simple offline "ora2xml" converter is available.

For development and evaluation purposes, COSMICrt also supports a raw logging system. When activated, all raw data along with the current timestamp in millisecond precision are saved to a local file. For efficiency reasons, this logging system makes use of the HDF5 format. HDF5 is short for "Hierarchical Data Format 5" and designed for the efficient storage of very large, mostly scientific, datasets. Libraries for all major programming languages are available, so that it is an easy task to read the data back using, for instance, a scripting language for evaluation purposes. See section 4.4 for details on how this was accomplished.

4.2.4. Control Loops

As soon as COSMICrt receives positional information from the MLC MCUs, one iteration of the control loop is run for the particular axis. The controllers are standard PID controllers as given by equation 2.4, but in their iterative form. The controllers themselves are integrated into the Control Thread of the COSMICrt application.

This iterated form is demonstrated in pseudo-code in listing 4.1. First, the parameters for the PID controller are set up and the current error (difference between target and current position) is calculated. Then, the time difference between last run of the control loop and current run is calculated.

The next step involves the calculation of integral and derivative and finally the gain based on the previous values.

As last step the current values for "integral" and "nError" are stored for the next run of the control loop.

```
1  fPIDKp = 0.4
2  fPIDKd = 0.003
3  fPIDKi = 0.005
4
5  nError = nCurrentPosition - nTargetPosition
6  dt = lastTimeStamp - thisTimeStamp
7
```

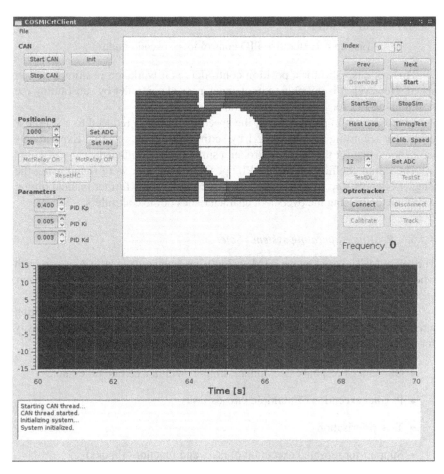

Figure 4.4: Main Screen of the COSMICrt control interface

```
 8 integral = (fPreIntegral + nError * dt)
 9 derivative = (nError - nPreError) / dt
10 gain = fPIDKp * nError + fPIDKi * integral + fPIDKd *
      derivative
11
12 fPreIntegral = integral
13 nPreError = nError
```

Listing 4.1: Iterative PID control loop; pseudo-code

This code is valid for a position controller, as it works on positions, not on speed. However, it is possible to implement a speed controller by substituting the positional values for "error" by speed values.

In the current implementation, the speed controller is reduced to a simple P controller according to equation 2.1 by setting K_I and K_D to zero. Experiments have shown that for the speed controller a simple gain is sufficient.

The initial coefficients for the PID position controller were found using the Ziegler-Nichols step response method. Afterwards, some further manual tuning was done, optimising the overshoot characteristics of the controllers.

4.2.5. Real-time operating system - Safety

The safety MCU, based on the ATMega2560, has some critical tasks to accomplish when it comes to safety and supervising of the whole system. For this reason, special care had to be taken in implementing this controller.

Originally, the safety system was implemented on the SORCUS SBC, running a real-time operating system (RTOS) called "OsX". The reasons and the necessity for a RTOS on this level are obvious (Tan and Anh 2009; Parikh et al. 2013):

- Guaranteed response to commands/inputs within a certain time range

- Parallel execution of multiple threads/tasks

- Task priorisation

- Support for repeated execution of tasks and functions (hooks)

- Better resource management

The need for an RTOS for the safety MCU was therefore given, but the choice of available RTOSs for the ATMega platform is very limited. This is also due to the fact that the ATMega features very low performance and has little RAM available. In the end, the choice for FreeRTOS was made based on a number of criteria. On the one hand, FreeRTOS has been on the market since at least 2004 (the Changelog misses the date entries for releases before 1.2.6) and since then has proved to be a stable and reliable operating system. On the other hand, it was ported to a number of microcontrollers, including the ATMega2560. Above all, a commercial implementation called SafeRTOS exists [8] which is SIL3 certified and can ultimately replace the open source version with only minimal changes to the current user level tasks involved.

Although executed on the Arduino platform, there is no Arduino code running on the safety MCU apart from the bootloader for easier programming.

The design implementation of the safety MCU consists of only two threads, namely the Ethernet Thread and the Interlock Thread. Both threads run on the FreeRTOS scheduler, but the priority of the Interlock Thread is higher than that of the Ethernet Thread.

The Ethernet Thread's responsibility is the communication with the control computer, respectively the control application. Once it receives the command to release the LinAc from the control application, it tells the Interlock Thread to release the LinAc. Thus, cross-thread communication capabilities are implemented on the RTOS.

The Interlock Thread continuously monitors the state of the MLC MCUs and reacts to their outputs. When they report an error, e.g. a mismatch between the two potentiometers, the LinAc is immediately stopped directly by the Interlock Thread.

Running on the RTOS, the advantage is guaranteed reaction time to any of the commands. A few instructions, mostly due to activity on the SPI bus, are non-interruptible, but apart from those critical tasks, a high-priority thread (Interlock Thread) can at any time interrupt the execution of the lower-priority thread (Ethernet Thread), if the time slice for higher-priority thread starts.

4.3. Test Setup

When all of the aforementioned subsystems are put together and configured correctly, irradiations using the realtime control system can be performed. In order to measure the performance of the complete system, a test setup was installed and a number of measurements, evaluating different characteristics of the system, were performed.

The tests were then carried out on the department's Elekta LinAc, in a simulated clinical environment.

---

[8]http://www.freertos.org, accessed Jan 2014

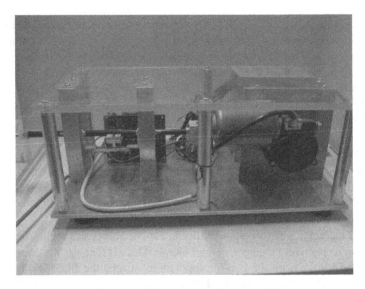

Figure 4.5: Picture of the in-house developed 4D phantom

4.3.1. 4D Phantom

For the simulation of a moving target, a 3D phantom, simulating e.g. a thorax, is
not sufficient. A 4D phantom, which also simulates the movements, is necessary.

A few years ago, a 4D phantom was developed in-house. To be precise, it is
a device that turns a 3D phantom into a 4D phantom, as it consists of a moving
carrier plate where any existing 3D phantom can be placed on.

Figure 4.5 (Böhler et al. 2015) depicts the 4D phantom, consisting of a carrier
plate (barely visible on the left), a motor and a power supply. As it turns a rotating
movement into a linear one, sinusoidal movements are the result. Speed adjustments
can be done using a potentiometer on the motor controller, two different amplitudes
can be adjusted by fixating the linear spindle on a different point on the rotating
wheel.

As it was implemented a few years back, no feedback or measurement system
was attached to the phantom. Therefore, the actual speed the phantom moves is
unknown and adjustments to the speed are trial and error. This renders the device
useless for measurements requiring knowledge of speed.

Because of this, a sliding potentiometer was attached to the linearly moving
part. This potentiometer can be powered and read by e.g. a microcontroller to

analyse the movement.

4.3.2. Artificial Tracking Signal

Another Arduino-based ATMega2560 was used to drive the potentiometer and read its values using the onboard AD converter. The raw values are then transferred via the universal serial bus (USB) to the control system, respectively the control application. Calibration and conversion to real world units is performed by COSMICrt inside the Phantom Thread.

Given the 10-bit AD converter on the ATMega, up to 1024 movement steps can be distinguished. For the phantom's drive length of 32 mm, this results in a resolution of 0.031 mm. For practical reasons, the two least significant bits were ignored, giving 256 steps resulting in a resolution of 0.125 mm.

On this MCU, another instance of FreeRTOS controls the reading of the values and the transfer to the control computer. Although this could have been implemented using interrupts as well, the RTOS makes software development easier without the need for setting up timers, interrupts and IO ports using low level instructions. Instead, the period length can be entered in physical units such as milliseconds.

4.3.3. Radiation Measurement

On this moving platform of the 4D phantom, a sandwich construction of a Gafchromic EBT2 film and solid water plates was placed (Butson et al. 2010; Cheung, Butson, and Yu 2006; García-Garduño et al. 2008). The film was put in maximum depth for 6 MV photons, which is 1.6 cm. The solid water plates are necessary for the secondary buildup that is responsible for achieving the maximum dose. The plates beneath the phantom serve the purpose of simulating back scattered photons from the surrounding tissue.

As the complete construction resides on the 4D phantom, it is moved along with the phantom. Therefore, the film always corresponds to the phantom's current positions that serve as input for the tracking system (as target positions).

4.3.4. MLC Setup

For measurement purposes, two MLCs need to be configured. This is on the one hand the LinAc's integrated MLC, the MLCi, and the add-on MLC containing the tracking field on the other. As the add-on MLC contains a moving field, the MLCi's field needs to be at least as large as the complete movement. To ease evaluation, the MLCi and the backup jaws were set to 10 cm by 12 cm in the isocentre, which

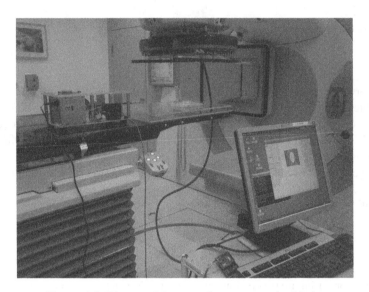

Figure 4.6: Picture of the complete setup at the LinAc

corresponds to the maximum field size of the Moduleaf miniMLC. The beam is thus, inside the measured areas, only collimated by the miniMLC.

Inside COSMICrt, a circular field with a diameter of 70 mm in the isocentre was loaded. This is the field shown in figure 4.4. The small open areas above and below the actual treatment field are the result of moving the leaves not involved in it as far outside as possible. They are usually covered by the MLCi and the backup jaws, just for this measurements the backup devices were moved out of the area.

200 Monitor Units (MU) of 6 MV photons were irradiated onto the phantom, corresponding to 2 Gy for a 10 cm by 10 cm field in maximum depth of 1.6 cm.

Figure 4.6 (Böhler et al. 2015) illustrates the complete setup at the LinAc. The computer in the foreground is the control computer, the 4D phantom is clearly visible on the couch.

Several measurements were performed with different motion settings. When measured in Hertz, evaluations were done for:

- Tracked Motion of 0.1 Hz, 0.2 Hz and 0.3 Hz

- Untracked Motion of 0.1 Hz, 0.25 Hz

The actual speed of the leaves and the 4D phantom depends on the amplitude of the sinusoidal movement, too. Taking the phantom's drive length of 32 mm

Frequency	Max. speed (isocentre)
0.1 Hz	20.1 mm/s
0.2 Hz	40.2 mm/s
0.25 Hz	50.25 mm/s
0.3 Hz	60.3 mm/s

Table 4.1: Comparison of phantom frequency and maximum leaf speed

into account, table 4.1 lists the maximum speed in the isocentre compared to the frequency.

This speed, the instantaneous speed, can be gained by derivating the sinusoidal function, visible in equation 4.1. By substituting the variables of the result, given in equation 4.2, the maximum speed can be found by setting $x = 0$.

$$\frac{\mathrm{d}}{\mathrm{d}x} 32 \sin\left(2 f_{Hz} \pi x\right) \tag{4.1}$$

$$64 f \pi \cos\left(2 f_{Hz} \pi x\right) \tag{4.2}$$

4.4. Data Analysis

In order to evaluate such a complex system, consisting of various subsystems, one measurement setup is not sufficient to characterise the system. The tracking accuracy has to be defined as well as the system's latency.

Two different types of measurement were performed simultaneously: timing and geometric accuracy. Both measurements have in common that as much raw data as possible was captured and analysed later on.

4.4.1. Timing Analysis

In order to be able to verify the timing and to measure the latency, all important internal numbers of COSMICrt were saved for analysis. Using the raw logging capabilities, the HDF5 file finally contained information on the current positions of the leaves, the current positions of the phantom and the target positions of the leaves. The timestamp that was saved along with each value has millisecond precision and presents an easy way to compare the signals. As all timestamps were generated by the same system, it is not necessary to synchronise clocks or to deal with drifting effects.

Furthermore, Linux uses the realtime clock only for the initial synchronisation with the system clock, but switches to a higher resolution timer as soon as possible. The acquired timestamps have at least microsecond precision, although nano seconds are reported. As this is not an RTOS, though, precision within the nano second league cannot be guaranteed (Gleixner and Niehaus 2006).

After performing the irradiation, the saved file was evaluated using a Python script. Python is a simple, yet powerful scripting language available for all common operating systems. It has libraries for nearly every file format and task available, including reading and manipulating HDF5 files.

The script first reads the data and corrects timestamps based on the initial offset. For comparing the signals, the raw data was resampled to 100 Hz using linear interpolation. Afterwards, the geometric error is calculated according to equation 4.3.

$$error = leafTargetPosition - leafCurrentPosition \qquad (4.3)$$

Cross correlating signals provides an easy means to calculate the time difference of the signals by virtually shifting one signals so that it aligns perfectly with the other signal. Equation 4.4 describes this cross correlation mathematically for the two signals f and g (Welch 1974).

$$(f \star g)[n] \stackrel{\text{def}}{=} \sum_{m=-\infty}^{\infty} f^*[m]\, g[n+m] \qquad (4.4)$$

The result of the cross correlation is again a function, where the index of the maximum value corresponds to the offset of the two input signals f and g.

For the creation of graphical representations, "matplotlib"[9] and "SciPy"[10] were used, both being scientific Python libraries.

4.4.2. Dose Measurements

In order to measure dose, the irradiated film has to be evaluated. As the response to irradiation of the film depends not only on the particular batch, but also on factors like age and exposure to sun light, each film needs to be calibrated beforehand.

Using FilmQA Pro 2013 (Ashland Advanced Materials, Bridgewater, USA), this calibration was performed before conducting the measurement. Afterwards, the irradiated film was scanned using an Epson scanner and imported into FilmQA Pro.

---

[9] http://matplotlib.org, accesssed Jan 2014
[10] scipy.org, accessed Jan 2014

Triple channel calibration was then performed, involving all three colour channels (Hayashi et al. 2012).

The central cross profile was selected and the absolute dose values were exported to a comma separated values (CSV) file for further analysis.

Again, a Python script was put in place that performed the actual analysis and comparison of the cross profiles. After the initial import into the Python script, the values were first normalised to the maximum, as only relative comparisons were performed. Then, the 20 % and 80 % threshold values were taken and the length of the penumbra was calculated, based on the known pixel density.

Again, plots were saved using "matploblib" and "SciPy".

5. Results

Results for both types of measurements, timing analysis and dose measurements, are described in this chapter.

5.1. Timing Analysis

The detailed results for each speed measurement are shown in figures 5.1 to 5.3. Only the results of the evaluation of one leaf – the central leaf with the widest opening – are shown. The red trace indicates the target leaf positions, the blue, triangled trace the leaf's current positions and the black, squared trace the geometric error according to equation 4.3. The traces for the leaf positions are shifted in the y-direction for better visiblity. All numbers are given in the isocentre plane whereas all traces are extracts from bigger datasets. Therefore, the x-axis and the timestamps do not start at zero, but rather at an arbitrary, high number.

The latency, determined by cross-correlating target positions and current positions, was determined to be 50 ms (window length 500 ms). It is the time introduced by the system from knowing the target position up to the reception of the leaf's current position. Although the latency stays about constant for different speeds, the actual shapes of the current positions do not. This is due to the limited leaf speed and the resulting geometrical error.

This value includes all aspects of the control application, MLC MCU system and mechanical components. The times to run the control loop, transfer the target position to the microcontroller, read the actual current position from the leaf and transfer the current position back to the control application are included.

The same figures show the geometrical error for each speed measurement, based on the reported current positions of the collimator system. It is shown that the geometrical error increases rapidly for faster speeds. As visible in figures 5.1 to 5.3, the geometrical error ranges from ± 2 mm for 0.1 Hz up to more than ± 15 mm for 0.3 Hz (Böhler et al. 2015).

Based on table 4.1, the maximum speed of the leaves for 0.1 Hz is 20 mm/s at the maximum, for 0.2 Hz this is 40 mm/s. A movement of 0.2 Hz is therefore at its maximum already faster than the leaves can travel (30 mm/s) (Schlegel et al. 2006).

This explains the bigger errors for faster movements than 0.2 Hz: The leaf simply cannot cope in time with the target position and, as a result, the error increases.

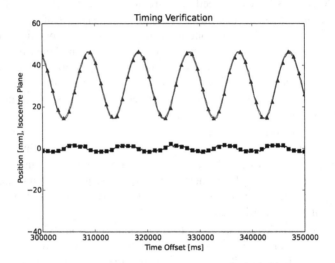

Figure 5.1: Positioning Error for 0.1 Hz; The straight line indicates the target position, the triangled line the current position and the squared line the positioning error. All numbers are in isocentre plane, current and target position have a constant offset for better visibility.

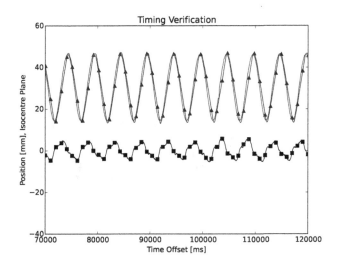

Figure 5.2: Positioning Error for 0.2 Hz; The straight line indicates the target position, the triangled line the current position and the squared line the positioning error. All numbers are in isocentre plane, current and target position have a constant offset for better visibility.

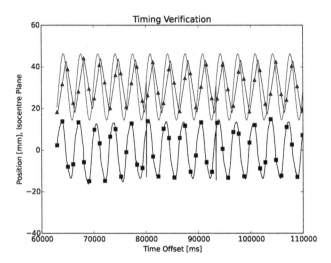

Figure 5.3: Positioning Error for 0.3 Hz; The straight line indicates the target position, the triangled line the current position and the squared line the positioning error. All numbers are in isocentre plane, current and target position have a constant offset for better visibility.

5.2. Dose Measurements

The geometric errors and latencies introduced by the control system have certain effects in terms of dose delivered to the target volume. Therefore, in combination with the timing evaluation, the dose irradiated onto the calibrated film was evaluated. In order to gain comparable results, the curves were normalised to the central axis. The penumbra width was then calculated by thresholding the data at 20 % and 80 %, respectively. The leaf pair with the widest opening, the same as in section 5.1, was chosen for calculating the penumbra.

Figures 5.4 to 5.6 show the individual penumbra widths and scanned films as measured by the application (Böhler et al. 2015). For comparison, an untracked penumbra as well as the digitised film are shown in figure 5.7 (Böhler et al. 2015). The red dots indicate the position of 20 % and 80 % dose, the penumbra is thus defined as the length between the respective two measurements points, projected onto the x-axis (the red sections, highlighted in green). By visually comparing the penumbra widths, there is no evident difference between figures 5.4 and 5.5. However, the visual shape of a penumbra taken by a phantom motion of 0.3 Hz (figure 5.6) differs from the previous two and tends towards the shape of an untracked phantom motion (figure 5.7).

The visual differences are confirmed by figure 5.8 (Böhler et al. 2015). There, the calculated penumbra widths are plotted against phantom motion. It is clearly visible that the penumbra width is only slighty widened for tracking speeds of up to 0.2 Hz. It tends rapidly towards very large penumbra widths that look like untracked penumbras for faster movements (blue, squared line). The latter, untracked penumbra widths are shown in figure 5.8 as well (green, dotted line).

For static fields, the Moduleaf's penumbra is less than 4 mm, thus the tracked penumbras for speeds of up to 0.2 Hz are only up to 1 mm wider (Solberg 2002).

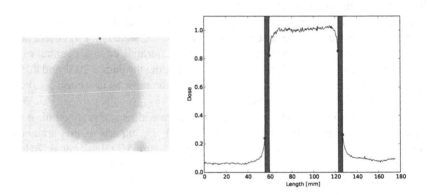

Figure 5.4: Penumbra Width for Phantom Motion of 0.1 Hz; the scanned, uncalibrated film is shown on the left, measured cross profile width on the right.

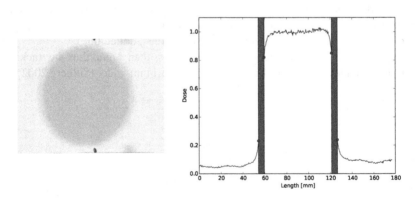

Figure 5.5: Penumbra Width for Phantom Motion of 0.2 Hz; the scanned, uncalibrated film is shown on the left, measured cross profile width on the right.

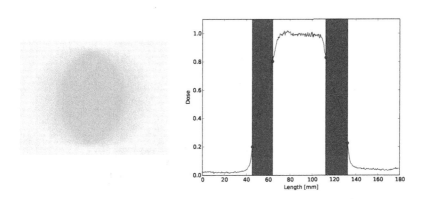

Figure 5.6: Penumbra Width for Phantom Motion of 0.3 Hz; the scanned, uncalibrated film is shown on the left, measured cross profile width on the right.

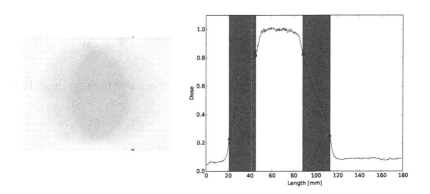

Figure 5.7: Penumbra Width of untracked Phantom Motion of 0.25 Hz; the scanned, uncalibrated film is shown on the left, measured cross profile width on the right.

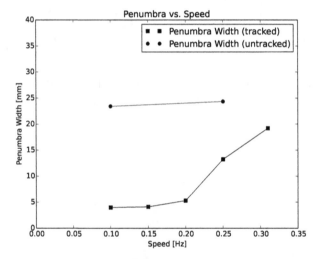

Figure 5.8: Comparison of Penumbra Widths: Tracked (squared line) vs. Untracked (dotted line)

6. Discussion

The Moduleaf miniMLC system was partially re-engineered and adapted to current treatment techniques. While only minor hardware modifications were made, the control software was completely redesigned from scratch.

Using open radART as PRVS, it is possible to use the Moduleaf as a DMLC, accepting field shape input from the PRVS and a further tracking signal input from other, external applications.

Analyses concerning the latency, the geometric error as well as the impact of those factors on the delivered dose were performed.

6.1. Methods

Concerning the methods, some improvements to the overall architecture and details can be made. It will further take some effort until the system can be turned into a medical device. Several of those aspects are discussed in the following chapters.

Although there is a safety system in place, consisting of an ATMega2560 MCU and interlock lines, it is not sufficient for patient safety. The RTOS running on this MCU is an open source system without any certification. However, there is also a commercial variant available which is certified and can be used for safety critical applications. In this case, also the hardware platform, the Arduino system, is an open source prototyping platform. Thus, it is equally difficult to certify the hardware according to medical standards. Several other aspects like housing for the MCU, cabling, etc. have to be dealt with as well.

The way the leaves are controlled in terms of data transfer and control loops was completely changed to host computer based data processing. While this significantly reduces the load of the individual MCUs, the host computer is under more pressure. COSMICrt was also developed using rapid prototyping techniques and a lot of open source software. While the same certification problems as with the open source hardware arises here, there are also some design limitations that would need to be reinvestigated.

The control software runs as a user space application. This means that the scheduler of the host operating system allocates CPU time to this and other applications according to the current scheduling algorithm. It therefore only has several time slices and other, high priority tasks could potentially interfere with the control system. This is no problem for the graphical user interface as it is non-critical, but the lower level systems such as the control loops and the digestion of the tracking input signal should be running with highest priorities. Realtime scheduling and a realtime kernel would therefore be preferred.

A possibility for achieving the separation and split of threads to realtime and non realtime threads would be the use of RTAI[1] and its extension called LXRT. RTAI (RealTime Application Interface) is an extension to the Linux kernel and provides realtime priorities, scheduler and realtime drivers for several devices. LXRT, on the other hand, provides realtime capabilities to user space applications. Therefore, parts of the COSMICrt threads could be implemented on LXRT and gain realtime capabilities. The certification problem, however, persists.

As few hardware modifications as possible were made to the system. Further hardware upgrades could potentially improve the system's performance. The leaf speed is currently limited by the maximum speed of the DC motors. An upgrade to the motors would improve speed and thus tracking performance (see also the discussion about the results in section 6.2 for more details).

Another performance improvement in terms of latency and feedback frequency could be achieved by replacing the MLC MCUs by faster variants. The current 16-bit MCUs running at 20 MHz significantly limit the number of interrupts per second and the amount of processing per second. Current XC167 MCUs, successors to the C167 platform, feature processing speeds of up to 40 MHz. Processing power is further improved by the use of a newer CPU design and the addition of a digital signal processor (DSP)[2].

The timing measurements as performed in section 4.4.1 compare the timing of individual subsystems. Usually, this requires accurate time synchronisation between the systems. In this case, however, all measurements were performed on the same computer, eliminating the synchronisation needs. The accuracy of the Linux high resolution timers in user space seem to be sufficiently high.

Real world signals usually differ from artificial signals used for evaluation purposes. In this case, the phantom simulated a steady, sinusoidal movement. However, a breathing cycle is not always steady. There is a sinusoidal movement involved, but after the exhalation, there is a short pause. As a sinusoidal movement was used, the type of motion seems valid. One advantage of the phantom is the ease with which knowledge about the current position can be gained. In real world, the tumour's motion has to be tracked with different methods. Examples for creating such a tracking signal include respiratory belts, X-Ray-based techniques, the RTRT system or surface scanners. Their latency, however, is in all cases bigger than the artificial tracking signal (Tetsuya Inoue et al. 2013; Krauss et al. 2012; Bibault et al. 2012; Harada et al. 2002; Poulsen, Cho, Sawant, and D. R. P. J. Keall 2010).

---

[1] http://www.rtai.org, accessed Jan 2014
[2] According to the XC167 datasheet

6.2. Results

Evaluations were performed for the geometric error, the system latency and the impact on dose. All measurements were conducted for different movement speeds.

Concerning latency, only the latency introduced by the control system was evaluated. The time the input system takes to generate the target position was not taken into account. Other apporaches to tracking, such as the upgraded Siemens 160-MLC, used image-based systems as inputs with high latencies of >400 ms (Tacke et al. 2010; Krauss et al. 2012).

The geometric accuracy of 2 mm for a maximum speed of 20 mm/s is worse than found in the literature with 1.1 mm for a maximum speed of about 10 mm/s (Paul J. Keall et al. 2006). As the speed is twice as high as in this work, the geometric accuracy for the slower speed should be on par with the literature. Furthermore, as mentioned before, the maximum leaf travel speed is limited by the DC motors.

Evaluations of the goemetric accuracy as well as the dosimetric impact were only performed for targets moving in the travel direction of the leaves. If the motion was not exactly aligned with the travel direction, the adjacent leaves would have to move very quickly in order to compensate the motion.

Dose measurements were performed on Gafchromic EBT2 film. It is suggested to calibrate each batch of the film, as calibration curves vary between batches (Mizuno et al. 2012). For this evaluation, only films of one batch, which was calibrated beforehand, were used. Furthermore, only relative comparisons between the measurements were conducted, thus eliminating inter film variations.

7. Conclusions

Given the technical limitations as discussed in section 6.1, the system is not yet ready for clinical use. The numbers, however, suggest that the device could be used for tracking applications within the limits of the system.

It is only usable for moving targets whose motions and diameter fit within the Moduleaf's treatment field of 10 cm by 12 cm in the isocentre. Furthermore, the system's characteristics are only known for movements within the leaf travel direction.

The tumour's motion should not exceed the maximum leaf travel speed of 30 mm/s. For faster moving targets, the leaves cannot catch up with the motion and penumbra widths are widened.

It was also shown that the measured penumbra width increases by 25 % for speeds of up to 0.2 Hz (40 mm/s) and increases rapidly for faster movements (>300 % for 0.3 Hz).

Using the system as a dynamic MLC for IMRT treatments, on the other hand, is another possible application. Here, the complete planning of the movement can be done in advance, taking into account the speed of the leaves and the limitations of the system. No realtime adaptations to the treatment field are necessary in this case.

All adaptations to the treatment field are calculated online in realtime. For, e.g., lung tumour tracking, the use of predictive algorithms can further improve tracking accuracy.

In combination with gating approaches, where the LinAc beam is simply stopped for a short period of time, the use of the system can be greatly improved. When the tumour motion is within the range of the MLC's capabilities, motion can be tracked and compensated for. If the tumour exceeds the MLC's capabilities, however, the gating interface would inhibit irradiation as long as necessary.

Even the combination of gating, DIBH and tracking would be feasible.

Bibliography

Ahmad, Saif S et al. (2012). "Advances in radiotherapy". In: *BMJ* 345. DOI: 10.1136/bmj.e7765.

Arjomandy, Bijan et al. (2012). "EBT2 film as a depth-dose measurement tool for radiotherapy beams over a wide range of energies and modalities". In: *Medical Physics* 39.2, pp. 912–921. DOI: 10.1118/1.3678989.

Åström, K.J. and T. Hägglund (1995). *PID controllers: Theory, design and tuning*. Research Triangle Park.

— (2001). "The future of PID control". In: *Control Engineering Practice* 9.11. PID Control, pp. 1163–1175. ISSN: 0967-0661. DOI: http://dx.doi.org/10.1016/S0967-0661(01)00062-4.

— (2004). "Revisiting the Ziegler–Nichols step response method for PID control". In: *Journal of Process Control* 14.6, pp. 635–650. ISSN: 0959-1524. DOI: http://dx.doi.org/10.1016/j.jprocont.2004.01.002.

Atherton, D.P. and S. Majhi (1999). "Limitations of PID controllers". In: *American Control Conference, 1999. Proceedings of the 1999*. Vol. 6, 3843–3847 vol.6. DOI: 10.1109/ACC.1999.786236.

Bedford, James, Michael Thomas, and Gregory Smyth (2013). "Beam modeling and VMAT performance with the Agility 160-leaf multileaf collimator". In: *Journal of Applied Clinical Medical Physics* 14.2, ISSN: 15269914.

Bibault, Jean-Emmanuel et al. (2012). "Image-Guided Robotic Stereotactic Radiation Therapy with Fiducial-Free Tumor Tracking for Lung Cancer". In: *Radiation Oncology* 7.1, p. 102. ISSN: 1748-717X. DOI: 10.1186/1748-717X-7-102.

Böhler, A et al. (2015). "Collimator based tracking with an add-on multileaf collimator: Moduleaf". In: *Physics in Medicine and Biology* 60.8, p. 3257. DOI: 10.1088/0031-9155/60/8/3257.

Bortfeld, Thomas, Steve B Jiang, and Eike Rietzel (2004). "Effects of motion on the total dose distribution". In: *Seminars in Radiation Oncology* 14.1, pp. 41–51. ISSN: 1053-4296. DOI: http://dx.doi.org/10.1053/j.semradonc.2003.10.011.

Boyer, Arthur et al. *AAPM Report No. 72: Basic Applications of Multileaf Collimators*. Tech. rep. Madison WI: American Association of Physicists in Medicine.

Butson, Martin J. et al. (2010). "Energy response of the new EBT2 radiochromic film to x-ray radiation". In: *Radiation Measurements* 45.7, pp. 836–839. ISSN: 1350-4487.

Cena, G. and A. Valenzano (2003). "Efficient polling of devices in CANopen networks". In: *Emerging Technologies and Factory Automation, 2003. Proceedings. ETFA '03. IEEE Conference*. Vol. 1, 123–130 vol.1. DOI: 10.1109/ETFA.2003.1247697.

Cheung, Tsang, Martin J. Butson, and Peter K. N. Yu (2006). "Measurement of high energy x-ray beam penumbra with Gafchromic EBT radiochromic film". In: *Medical Physics* 33.8, pp. 2912–2914. DOI: 10.1118/1.2218318.

Crop, F et al. (2007). "Monte Carlo modeling of the ModuLeaf miniature MLC for small field dosimetry and quality assurance of the clinical treatment planning system". In: *Physics in Medicine and Biology* 52.11, p. 3275.

Delaney, Geoff et al. (2005). "The role of radiotherapy in cancer treatment". In: *Cancer* 104.6, pp. 1129–1137. ISSN: 1097-0142. DOI: 10.1002/cncr.21324.

Falk, Marianne et al. (2010). "Real-time dynamic MLC tracking for inversely optimized arc radiotherapy." In: *Radiother Oncol* 94.2, pp. 218–23. DOI: 10.1016/j.radonc.2009.12.022.

Farsi, M. and K. Ratcliff (1997). "An introduction to CANopen and CANopen communication issues". In: *CANopen Implementation (Digest No. 1997/384), IEE Colloquium on*, pp. 2/1–2/6. DOI: 10.1049/ic:19971322.

Farsi, M., K. Ratcliff, and M. Barbosa (1999a). "An introduction to CANopen". In: *Computing Control Engineering Journal* 10.4, pp. 161–168. ISSN: 0956-3385. DOI: 10.1049/cce:19990405.

— (1999b). "An overview of controller area network". In: *Computing Control Engineering Journal* 10.3, pp. 113–120. ISSN: 0956-3385. DOI: 10.1049/cce:19990304.

Gaisberger, C. et al. (2013). "Three-dimensional surface scanning for accurate patient positioning and monitoring during breast cancer radiotherapy". English. In: *Strahlentherapie und Onkologie* 189.10, pp. 887–893. ISSN: 0179-7158. DOI: 10.1007/s00066-013-0358-6.

García-Garduño, Olivia Amanda et al. (2008). "Radiation transmission, leakage and beam penumbra measurements of a micro-multileaf collimator using GafChromic EBT film." In: *J Appl Clin Med Phys* 9.3, p. 2802.

Geoffrey, G et al. (2012). "Motion Management in Stereotactic Body Radiotherapy". In: *Journal of Nuclear Medicine & Radiation Therapy*.

Gleixner, Thomas and Douglas Niehaus (2006). "Hrtimers and beyond: Transforming the linux time subsystems". In: *Linux Symposium*. Vol. 1. Citeseer, pp. 333–346.

Guckenberger, Matthias et al. (2009). "Potential of image-guidance, gating and real-time tracking to improve accuracy in pulmonary stereotactic body radiotherapy". In: *Radiotherapy and oncology : journal of the European Society for Therapeutic Radiology and Oncology, Radiother Oncol* 91.3, pp. 288–295. ISSN: 0167-8140.

Harada, Toshiyuki et al. (2002). "Real-time tumor-tracking radiation therapy for lung carcinoma by the aid of insertion of a gold marker using bronchofiberscopy". In: *Cancer* 95.8, pp. 1720–1727. ISSN: 1097-0142. DOI: 10.1002/cncr.10856.

Hayashi, Naoki et al. (2012). "Evaluation of triple channel correction acquisition method for radiochromic film dosimetry". In: *Journal of Radiation Research* 53.6, pp. 930–935. DOI: 10.1093/jrr/rrs030. eprint: http://jrr.oxfordjournals.org/content/53/6/930.full.pdf+html.

Herk, Marcel van (2004). "Errors and margins in radiotherapy". In: *Seminars in radiation oncology, Semin Radiat Oncol* 14.1, pp. 52–64. ISSN: 1053-4296.

Hoogeman, Mischa et al. (2009). "Clinical Accuracy of the Respiratory Tumor Tracking System of the CyberKnife: Assessment by Analysis of Log Files". In: *Int J Radiat Oncol Biol Phys* 74.1, pp. 297–303. ISSN: 0360-3016.

Ikushima, Hitoshi (2010). "Radiation therapy: state of the art and the future". In: *The Journal of Medical Investigation* 57.1,2, pp. 1–11.

Inoue, Tetsuya et al. (2013). "Stereotactic body radiotherapy using gated radiotherapy with real-time tumor-tracking for stage I non-small cell lung cancer". In: *Radiation Oncology* 8.1, p. 69. ISSN: 1748-717X. DOI: 10.1186/1748-717X-8-69.

Inoue, T. et al. (2013). "Stereotactic body radiotherapy for pulmonary metastases". English. In: *Strahlentherapie und Onkologie* 189.4, pp. 285–292. ISSN: 0179-7158. DOI: 10.1007/s00066-012-0290-1.

Jereczek-Fossa, B.A. et al. (2013). "CyberKnife robotic image-guided stereotactic radiotherapy for oligometastic cancer". English. In: *Strahlentherapie und Onkologie* 189.6, pp. 448–455. ISSN: 0179-7158. DOI: 10.1007/s00066-013-0345-y.

Jiang, Steve B. (2006). "Medical dosimetry : official journal of the American Association of Medical Dosimetrists". In: 31.2, pp. 141–151. ISSN: 0958-3947.

Keall, Paul J. et al. (2006). "Geometric accuracy of a real-time target tracking system with dynamic multileaf collimator tracking system". In: *International journal of radiation oncology, biology, physics* 65.5, pp. 1579–1584. ISSN: 0360-3016.

Knoll, G.F. (2010). *Radiation Detection and Measurement*. John Wiley & Sons. ISBN: 9780470131480.

Krauss, Andreas et al. (2012). "Multileaf collimator tracking integrated with a novel x-ray imaging system and external surrogate monitoring". In: *Physics in Medicine and Biology* 57.8, p. 2425.

Kubo, Hideo D and Bruce C Hill (1996). "Respiration gated radiotherapy treatment: a technical study". In: *Physics in Medicine and Biology* 41.1, p. 83.

Laub, Wolfram U. and Tony Wong (2003). "The volume effect of detectors in the dosimetry of small fields used in IMRT". In: *Medical Physics* 30.3, pp. 341–347. DOI: http://dx.doi.org/10.1118/1.1544678.

Liu, G.P. and S. Daley (2001). "Optimal-tuning PID control for industrial systems". In: *Control Engineering Practice* 9.11. PID Control, pp. 1185–1194. ISSN: 0967-0661. DOI: http://dx.doi.org/10.1016/S0967-0661(01)00064-8.

Mackie, T. Rockwell et al. (1999). "Tomotherapy". In: *Seminars in Radiation Oncology* 9.1. Radiation Therapy Treatment Optimization, pp. 108–117. ISSN: 1053-4296. DOI: http://dx.doi.org/10.1016/S1053-4296(99)80058-7.

Mageras, Gikas S and Ellen Yorke (2004). "Deep inspiration breath hold and respiratory gating strategies for reducing organ motion in radiation treatment". In: *Seminars in Radiation Oncology* 14.1. <ce:title>High-Precision Radiation Therapy of Moving Targets</ce:title>, pp. 65–75. ISSN: 1053-4296. DOI: http://dx.doi.org/10.1053/j.semradonc.2003.10.009.

McMahon, Ryan, Lech Papiez, and Dharanipathy Rangaraj (2007). "Dynamic-MLC leaf control utilizing on-flight intensity calculations: A robust method for real-time IMRT delivery over moving rigid targets". In: *Medical Physics* 34.8. DOI: 10.1118/1.2750964.

Mizuno, Hirokazu et al. (2012). "Homogeneity of GAFCHROMIC EBT2 film among different lot numbers". In: *Journal of Applied Clinical Medical Physics* 13.4. ISSN: 15269914.

Mzenda, Bongile et al. (2010). "A simulation technique for computation of the dosimetric effects of setup, organ motion and delineation uncertainties in radiotherapy". English. In: *Medical & Biological Engineering & Computing* 48.7, pp. 661–669. ISSN: 0140-0118. DOI: 10.1007/s11517-010-0616-z.

Paliwal, Bhudatt. and Dinesh. Tewatia (2009). "Advances in radiation therapy dosimetry". In: *Journal of Medical Physics* 34.3, pp. 108–116. DOI: 10.4103/0971-6203.54842.

Parikh, H. et al. (2013). "Performance parameters of RTOSs; comparison of open source RTOSs and benchmarking techniques". In: *Advances in Technology and Engineering (ICATE), 2013 International Conference on*, pp. 1–6. DOI: 10.1109/icadte.2013.6524742.

Pfeiffer, O., A. Ayre, and C. Keydel (2008). *Embedded Networking with CAN and CANopen*. Copperhill Technologies Corporation. ISBN: 9780976511625.

Pinho, L.M. and F. Vasques (2003). "Reliable real-time communication in CAN networks". In: *Computers, IEEE Transactions on* 52.12, pp. 1594–1607. ISSN: 0018-9340. DOI: 10.1109/TC.2003.1252855.

Poulsen, Per Rugaard, Byungchul Cho, Amit Sawant, and Dan Ruan Paul J Keall (2010). "Detailed analysis of latencies in image-based dynamic MLC tracking". In: *Medical Physics* 37.9. DOI: 10.1118/1.3480504.

Poulsen, Per Rugaard, Byungchul Cho, Amit Sawant, and Paul J Keall (2010). "Implementation of a new method for dynamic multileaf collimator tracking of prostate motion in arc radiotherapy using a single kV imager." In: *Int. J. Radiat. Oncol. Biol. Phys.* 76.3, pp. 914–23. DOI: 10.1016/j.ijrobp.2009.06.073.

Sawant, Amit et al. (2008). "Management of three-dimensional intrafraction motion through real-time DMLC tracking". In: *Medical Physics* 35.5, pp. 2050–2061. DOI: http://dx.doi.org/10.1118/1.2905355.

Schlegel, W.C. et al. (2006). *New Technologies in Radiation Oncology*. Medical Radiology. Springer. ISBN: 9783540299998.

Solberg, Timothy (2002). "Field Shaping; Design Characteristics and Dosimetry Issues". In: *44th AAPM Annual Meeting*.

Tacke, Martin B. et al. (2010). "Real-time tumor tracking: Automatic compensation of target motion using the Siemens 160 MLC". In: *Medical Physics* 37.2, pp. 753–761. DOI: http://dx.doi.org/10.1118/1.3284543.

Tan, Su-Lim and Tran Nguyen Bao Anh (2009). "Real-time operating system (RTOS) for small (16-bit) microcontroller". In: *Consumer Electronics, 2009. ISCE '09. IEEE 13th International Symposium on*, pp. 1007–1011. DOI: 10.1109/ISCE.2009.5156833.

Tindell, K. W., H. Hansson, and A. J. Wellings (1994). "Analysing real-time communications: controller area network (CAN)". In: *Real-Time Systems Symposium, 1994., Proceedings*. Pp. 259–263. DOI: 10.1109/real.1994.342710.

Trofimov, Alexei et al. (2008). "Tumor trailing strategy for intensity-modulated radiation therapy of moving targets". In: *Medical Physics* 35.5, pp. 1718–1733. DOI: http://dx.doi.org/10.1118/1.2900108.

Vedam, S. S. et al. (2001). "Determining parameters for respiration-gated radiotherapy". In: *Medical Physics* 28.10, pp. 2139–2146. DOI: http://dx.doi.org/10.1118/1.1406524.

Voort van Zyp, Noëlle C. van der et al. (2009). "Stereotactic radiotherapy with real-time tumor tracking for non-small cell lung cancer: Clinical outcome". In: *Radiotherapy and oncology : journal of the European Society for Therapeutic Radiology and Oncology, Radiother Oncol* 91.3, pp. 296–300. ISSN: 0167-8140.

Welch, L. (1974). "Lower bounds on the maximum cross correlation of signals (Corresp.)" In: *Information Theory, IEEE Transactions on* 20.3, pp. 397–399. ISSN: 0018-9448. DOI: 10.1109/TIT.1974.1055219.

Wu, Q Jackie et al. (2009). "Impact of collimator leaf width and treatment technique on stereotactic radiosurgery and radiotherapy plans for intra- and extracranial lesions". In: *Radiation Oncology* 4.1, p. 3. ISSN: 1748-717X. DOI: 10.1186/1748-717x-4-3.

Yime, Eugenio (2008). "CAN on Parallel Robots: How to Control a Stewart Platform using CAN based motor controllers". In: *Proceedings of the 12th iCC 2008*.

Ziouva, Eustathia and Theodore Antonakopoulos (2002). "CSMA/CA performance under high traffic conditions: throughput and delay analysis". In: *Computer Communications* 25.3, pp. 313–321.

Printed in the United States
By Bookmasters